Health Benefits of Black Cumin

For Cooking and Health

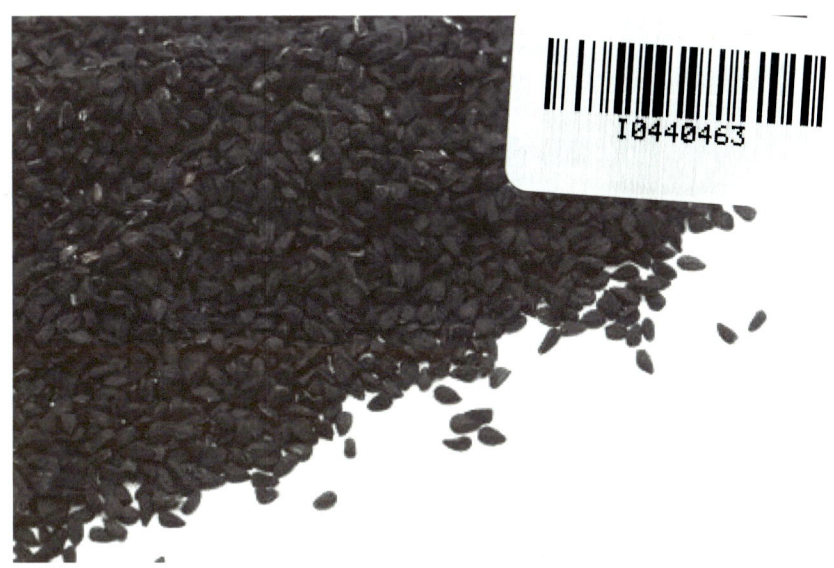

By M.Usman

Health Learning Series

Mendon Cottage Books

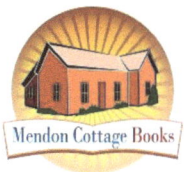

JD-Biz Publishing

Download Free Books!

http://MendonCottageBooks.com

All Rights Reserved.

No part of this publication may be reproduced in any form or by any means, including scanning, photocopying, or otherwise without prior written permission from JD-Biz Corp Copyright © 2015
All Images Licensed by Fotolia and 123RF

Disclaimer

The information is this book is provided for informational purposes only. It is not intended to be used and medical advice or a substitute for proper medical treatment by a qualified health care provider. The information is believed to be accurate as presented based on research by the author.

The contents have not been evaluated by the U.S. Food and Drug Administration or any other Government or Health Organization and the contents in this book are not to be used to treat cure or prevent disease or mental illness.

The author or publisher is not responsible for the use or safety of any diet, procedure or treatment mentioned in this book. The author or publisher is not responsible for errors or omissions that may exist.

Warning

The Book is for informational purposes only and before taking on any diet, treatment or medical procedure it is recommended to consult with your primary care provider.

Our books are available at

1. Amazon.com
2. Barnes and Noble
3. Itunes
4. Kobo
5. Smashwords
6. Google Play Books

Table of Contents

Preface

Many plants that seem so innocuous to us today have been used in traditional medicine for centuries and have produced astonishing results. Greek and Indian medicine in particular has taken leverage of numerous herbs and plants in curing a wide variety of ailments. Only today has science caught up with what our ancestors took as common knowledge. Research conducted over the past few decades have begun to testify to the health benefits of these botanical wonders.

One such amazing plant is Black Cumin more specifically known as Nigella sativa. It is a plant that blossoms yearly and was found originally in the southern and southwestern regions of Asia. Growing to a height ranging from twenty to thirty centimeters, it is characterized by its thin and straight leaves, fragile blue / white flowers and large bloated fruit holding the renowned Black Cumin seed.

The seed of this plant has been used in cuisines around the globe but is particularly famous and notable in Sub-continental cooking. Its pungent taste and unique aroma has made it famous in many dishes. Its importance in the kitchen aside, this seed has a host of medicinal benefits that make it ideal for consumption from a health perspective. It can have a positive effect on both body and mind and scientific evidence has been gathered to support this.

This book aims to educate you in the many benefits of this truly miraculous plant whose seeds work wonders for human health. It will instruct you on the best way to take advantage of Black Cumin's benefits and easily make it a part of your daily life. There will also be tips on cultivating your own Black Cumin seeds to use in your kitchen! By the time you reach the end, this humble plant will have definitely made an impression on your mind.

Many of you will have overlooked Black Cumin seeds as a mere spice to be used in cooking but after reading the health benefits of the same, you'll begin to look at them with a new found reverence.

Getting Started

Chapter # 1: Intro

Before delving into the numerous benefits of Black Cumin, it is a good idea to become acquainted with the basic information concerning this plant.

Identifying traits

Black cumin, scientifically known as Nigella sativa, is a plant that blooms every year and originated in the south and south-west of Asia. It is identifiable by its height ranging from 8 to 12 inches, it's linear, thinly cut leaves, its soft flowers that are a shade of either blue or white, and its large, bloated capsule like fruit which is filled with its seeds- The same seeds that are found in kitchens around the globe as spice.

Etymology

Its scientific name, Nigella Sativa, was derived from the Latin word 'Niger' meaning black – a reference to the black color of its seeds.

Many names have been given to the plant and its seeds. The English have called it by monikers such as fennel flower, nutmeg flower, black caraway and Roman coriander. And of course, black cumin has been the most popular name given to. There has also been some mistaken etymology concerning this plant where it has been wrongly called onion seed or black sesame, which bear a resemblance but are completely different seeds.

Some of the names given to the seeds by various cultures include *kalijeera* (Assamese), *kalo jire* (Bengali), *habbat al-barakah* (Arabic), *reske* (Kurdish), *kalonji* or *kalaunji* (Urdu / Hindi), *mangrail* (Hindi), *ketzakh* (Hebrew), *chernushka* (Russian), *çörek otu* (Turkish), *siyahdaneh* (Persian), *jintan hitam* (Indonesian), *karim jeerakam* (Malayalam) etc.

Chemistry

The oil extracted from Black Cumin seeds is composed of:

- conjugated linoleic acid
- thymoquinone
- nigellone
- melanthin
- nigilline
- damascenine
- tannins

History

Nigella sativa seeds were found in the tomb of the ancient Egyptian emperor Tutankhamun. Although the exact degree of the Egyptians awareness of the benefits of this plant has not been determined, this does imply that ancient Egyptians were aware of some of its virtues which is why it was placed to assist the pharaoh in the afterlife.

It is also mentioned in words in the Old Testament and was found in a vessel in Turkey that dated two thousand years BC.

Chapter # 2: How is black cumin commonly used?

Uses in cuisine

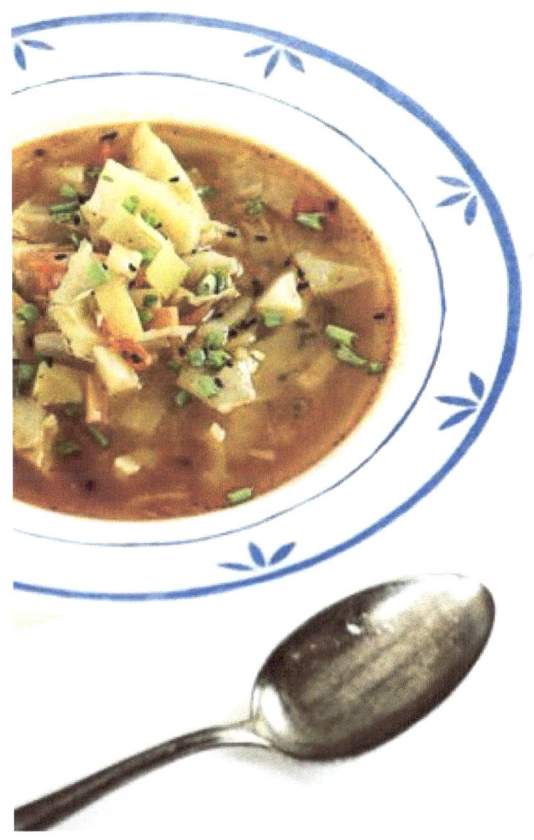

It enjoys a unique position in the cuisine of many counties by virtue of its sharp bitter taste and aroma:

In Bengali cooking, it mixed with four other spices to make *panch phoran* that is used in a good number of Bengali dishes. It is also used on its own in several dishes; a notable example is the famous naan bread.

In Turkey, too, it is used in the renowned *çörek* buns as a flavoring and in Bosnia; it is used as a flavor in pastries that are frequently baked on Islamic religious occasions. This is particularly common in the capital city of Sarajevo. The well-known Peshawari naan employ it as a topping.

The diversity of its cooking applications is such that it makes its way in string cheeses made in Armenia and the Middle East!

Uses in traditional medicine

As already mentioned Black Cumin is an integral medicinal plant in Greek medicine and is claimed to fight a sizeable number of diseases.

People belonging to the regions of the Middle East and South Asia have used it to treat respiratory conditions such as a blocked nose where the effect of its aroma has been compared to that of crushed eucalyptus leaves.

Research that has been conducted into the medicinal effects of black cumin in recent years has begun to yield evidence to support its importance in traditional medicine.

There has been some controversy that Nestlé has filed an application for patenting one of the core constituents of black cumin oil i.e.

thymoquinone. This move has been met by widespread criticism from alternate and herbal health enthusiasts who claim that the firm is trying to limit the access of people to this plant. Whatever the truth maybe, it is clear that black cumin must be of some import to merit a patent application from a firm as big as Nestlé.

Chapter # 3: Black cumin recipes

It has already been stated that black cumin is used in a great deal of foods around the world to lend a special taste and smell to them. Below are detailed some particularly tasty recipes that make use of this spice and will not only make your food tastier but also healthier.

Mirchi Ka Salan (Hyderabadi cuisine):

This is a recipe to a spicy all vegan dish that is sure to pack a punch at any dinner.

Ingredients:

200 g long **green chilies**

1 tsp **cumin seeds**

1/2 tsp **mustard seeds**

1/4 tsp **fenugreek seeds**

1/4 tsp **nigella seeds**

6 **curry leaves**

1/4 tsp **turmeric powder**

2 tbsp. **coriander-cumin seeds powder**

2 tsp **chili powder**

4 tbsp. **Tamarind water**

2 tbsp. **Chopped coriander**

5 tbsp. **oil**

salt to taste

[Make into a paste]

6 cloves of **garlic**

12 mm. (1/2") piece **ginger**

1 **onion**

2 **tomatoes**

3 tbsp. **grated coconut**

[Grind into a dry powder]

2 tbsp. **Roasted peanuts**

2 tbsp. **sesame seeds**

1 tbsp. **cumin seeds**

Procedure:

[To make the dry powder]

Roast the ingredients lightly then remove and grind to a powder.

[To cook the dish]

Heat oil in a metal *karahi* and while this happens, wash and slit the green chilies to remove their seeds after which you should fry them in the now hot until they turn a color of white.

Next add the cumin, fenugreek, mustard and nigella seeds, and curry leaves into the same oil (after taking out the chilies). Cook the mixture until the seeds start crackling.

Now add the paste you made earlier and fry for some time. Following this, put in the turmeric and coriander-cumin seed mix, the chill powder and the dry powder that was also prepared previously. Cook this new mixture for some minutes up to the point that the oil envelops them.

Next pour in two cups of water, and the tamarind juice and cook to make thick gravy like texture. Add the fried chilies, coriander and salt at this point as well.

Serve while hot and enjoy.

Nigella sativa power honey mixture:

This is a recipe for an extremely nutritious and potent mixture that can be used as a dietary supplement to keep you charged throughout the day. The sweet taste and smooth texture of the honey make this power mixture a treat for the taste buds too!

Ingredients

3 cups honey

2 tbsp. Royal honey

2 tbsp. Nigella sativa seeds + oil

2 tbsp. Ginger powder

1/3 cup chopped nuts [almonds, pistachios preferred)

Procedure

Put the honey, seeds and ginger into a medium bowl and mix them up. For the black cumin part of the mixture, it is up to your discretion to use seeds or oil. Oil is chosen by some for its consistency. In any case, the seeds must be heat before they are put into the mixture.

After the honey mixture is ready, put in the chopped nuts. The resulting power mixture should be stored in sealed vessels and can be used to sweeten foods or directly as a daily power booster.

Khobz Mzaweq (Moroccan bread):

With so much importance given to black cumin as an ingredient in making various breads and baked goods, this section will be concluded with a recipe for making a delicious and filling bread baked in Morocco which contains sesame, semolina and black cumin seeds.

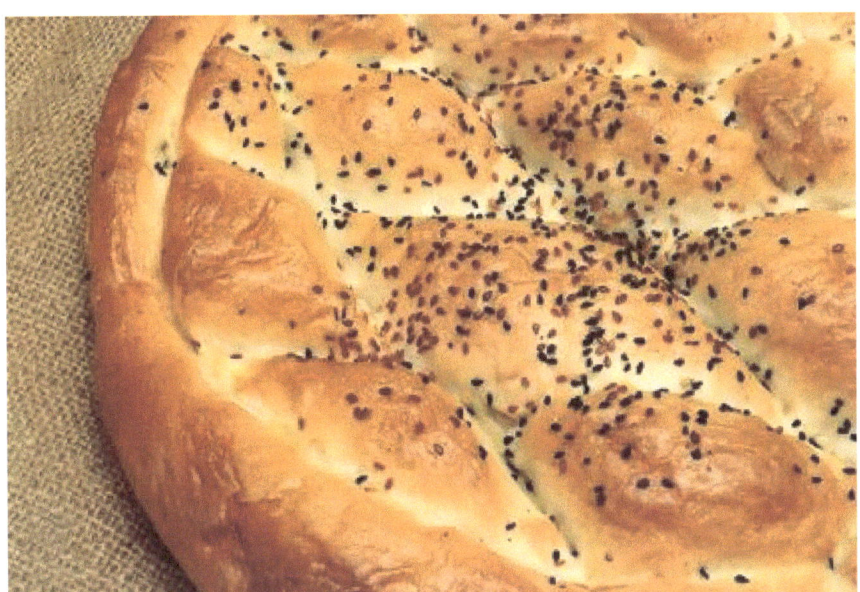

The reasoning behind its name which literally means decorated bread is that its top is decorated with a crisscrossing pattern after which is garnished with egg yolk and sprinkled with more seeds.

This bread gives you a lot of room for experimentation by changing the ratios of various ingredients and is ideally suited for serving at breakfast or tea. Sandwiches made from it are equally delicious.

Ingredients

2 1/2 cups white flour

1 1/2 cups fine semolina flour

1 tbsp. sugar

2 tsp. salt

2 tsp. sesame seeds

2 tsp. nigella seeds

1 tbsp. yeast

2 tbsp. vegetable oil

1 egg

1 cup (approx.) warm water

additional flour for kneading

semolina flour or oil for the pan

[For the garnish]

1 egg yolk, lightly beaten

1 to 2 tsp. sesame seeds

Procedure

The sheet used for baking should be prepped by oiling its center or by sprinkling the pan with some semolina flour.

The dry ingredients should be mixed in a bowl following which a large well shaped hole should be made in the center of the mix. The egg, yeast, oil and water should be put in next. The wet ingredients should be mixed to dissolve the yeast and then the full contents in the bowl should be mixed too, so that the dry and wet ingredients can combine properly.

This dough should be turned on a surface sprinkled with flour and then kneaded. Water and flour should be added as required on the dough to make sure that it remains soft and tender, and does not stick. This kneading should continue for about ten minutes or as long as the dough hasn't turned elastic and smooth, whichever comes first.

The dough should then be made into a level and round mound and put on to the baking pan prepared earlier. It should then be covered with a kitchen towel and rested for some fifteen minutes.

Once the dough is rested, it should be flattened into a circle with a thickness of a quarter inch by using the palm of the hand. It should again be covered with the towel and left for around an hour to rise. The condition is that the dough becomes springy when pressed.

The oven should be preheated to 435 degrees Fahrenheit / 225 degrees Celsius.

Now the towel should be removed and the diamond shaped patterns made on it by means of a sharp knife. It should then be garnished with egg yolk and sesame seeds and baked for around twenty to twenty five minutes. You'll know when to stop when the bread turns a rich color and emits a hollow sound when tapped. The bread can then be put onto a rack or a basket lined with towels to cool down.

At room temperature, this bread keeps fresh for a day but when frozen, it can keep for a month!

Chapter # 4: Growing your own black cumin

Although nigella sativa is best grown in its natural habitat, it is possible to grow it in your own garden if you so desire.

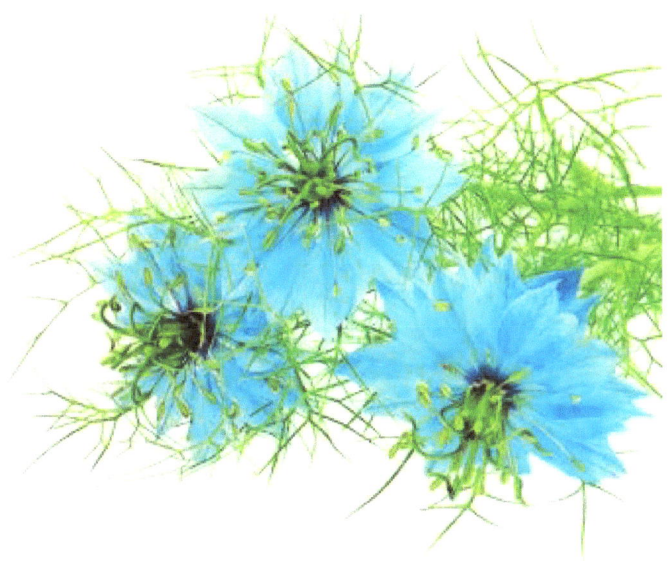

The planting should be done in November before the first frost sets in when grown outdoors. It may also be planted in peat pots to be grown indoors but in this case, the planting should be done before the onset of autumn or spring, and then the plants should be transplanted in the garden.

The rows in which the planting is done should be separated by a foot and the soil must contain ample water. It will take two weeks for the seeds to show signs of germination when grown outside from the start. The peat pots take some seven weeks to germinate and become ready for transplantation.

Once the flowers have blossomed, the black cumin pods should be removed and placed in brown paper bags to dry up and the bags then rubbed with the hands to extract the seeds. A cut can be made in a corner of the bag to let the seeds trickle into a filter so that any waste material is removed.

The seeds should be dried completely and then placed in a sealed jar for storage.

Chapter # 5: Precautions

Black cumin, when taken in excess of 25 grams, can be toxic but this amount is truly abnormal since the maximum dosage for any medicinal treatment involving black cumin is 3 tablespoons a day. You should not fall for any sight that tries to sell black cumin seed or oil on the principle of more is better.

Black cumin oil should not be consumed with a full stomach and must be mixed with another liquid to such as a juice, some yogurt or honey. One hour before any meal will do the trick.

The seeds should be heated before consumption to avoid upsetting the stomach.

Additionally, pregnant women and those suffering from blood pressure dependent conditions should avoid using black cumin seeds.

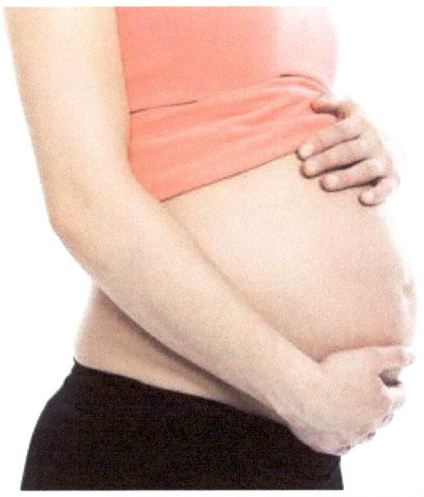

Benefits of black cumin to the brain

Chapter # 6: Boosts memory

The Journal of Ethno pharmacology, in one of its publications, highlighted the brain enhancing properties of black cumin.

According to the study, 20 men in their fifties who took 2 500mg doses of pure black seed in the form capsules holding ground black seed powder each day for 9 weeks, showed decidedly better performance in terms of memory, attention span and cognition compared to their control counterparts.

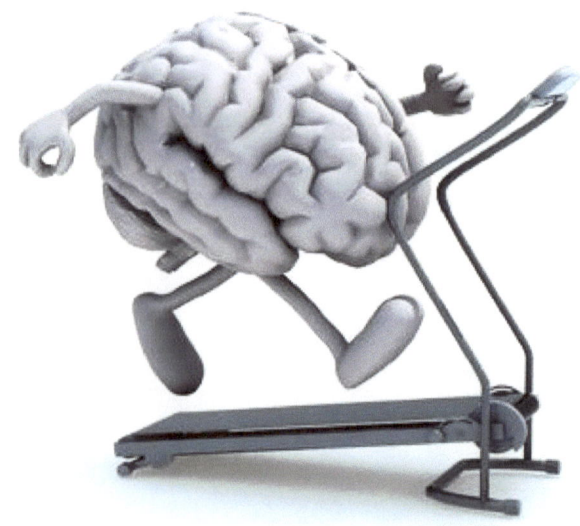

It has been suggested by Muhammad Shahdaat Bin Sayeed, a lecturer of pharmacy at the University of Asia Pacific in Bangladesh and the writer of the study, that black cumin's abilities to bar oxidation, inflammation and damage to neurons in the body are accountable for the brain enhancing results.

The abundance of essential oils, known for giving stimulus to the brain, in black cumin can be a factor in the brain improving results as well since it stoppers the disintegration of neurotransmitters, an established approach to bettering memory function. When these neurotransmitters are destroyed, our normal memory function is adversely effected says the author of the study; black seed has the property to stop this degradation of neurotransmitters.

Major human organs such as the heart, liver and kidney did not suffer from any side effects due to the consumption of black cumin during the study which means that it is safe for supplemental consumption.

Although black cumin has not become popular as a pharmaceutical drug yet, it can be used by coupling it with some honey or mint to make its sharp flavor easier on the taste buds.

Black cumin shows a lot of promise as a brain boosting spice.

Benefits of black cumin to the body

Chapter # 7: Fights cancer

Black cumin's ability to fight cancer has been tested and proven by numerous studies conducted by reputed organizations.

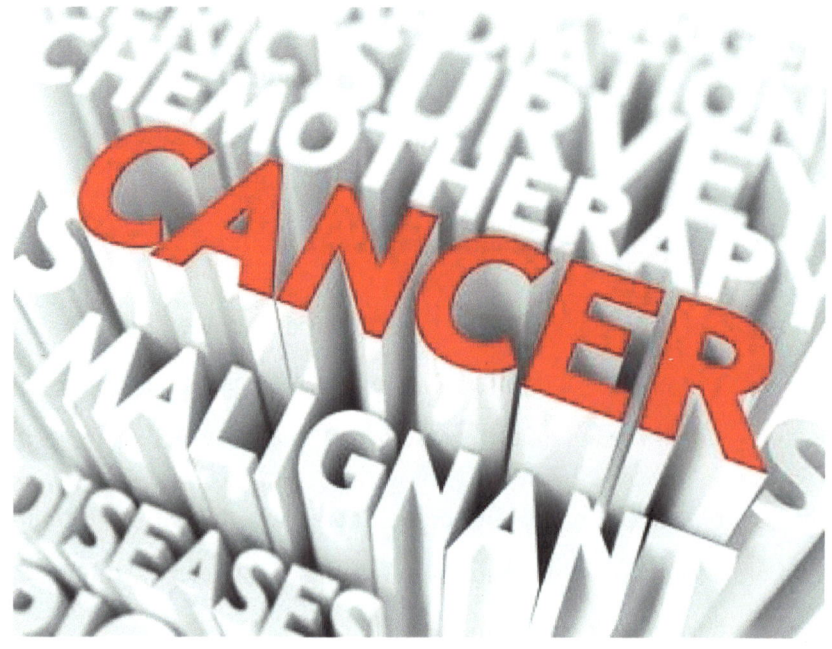

Its ability to destroy cancer cells was tested by researchers at Kimmel Cancer Center at Jefferson where the results clearly illustrated that nigella sativa could kill pancreatic tumor cells. The success rate was found to be a good 80% and many future studies seem to be in order following the success of this research.

Hwyda Arafat, an associate professor of Surgery at the College of Thomas Jefferson University says that previous studies on black cumin have revealed an ability to fight prostate and colon cancers as well. Its effect on breast cancer has also been studied by other research groups and these studies have shown a remarkable proficiency of black seed in ensuring good health among women.

Additionally, there have been numerous testimonies by individuals who claim that their cancers have been miraculously cured by the use of black cumin. The cancers were diverse including brain, bone and stomach cancer.

According to the Cancer Research Laboratory of Hilton Head Island, South Carolina, USA, considerable success was found in the treatment of tumors by black cumin minus the side effects of chemo. The use of black cumin speeded up the growth of bone marrow cells by an astounding 250 percent and limited the growth of the tumor by half. This was linked to black cumin's ability to boost the immune system by raising the production of interferon. By doing this, the black cumin oil enables the immune system to destroy the cancer cells before they become a problem for the person.

For those who have trouble understanding, here is a simple explanation of how black cumin seed oil helps fight cancer. They contain an active component in their oil called *thymoquinone*. This compound improves the survival and working of key cells in the immune system of the body. These cells are called T-cells.

These cells can be thought of as the body's first response team against cancerous cells that, after deployment by the help of certain other cells, track down and eliminate cancer cells. This whole exercise of the deployment of T-cells by helper cells is known as 'conditioning'and it increases their efficiency against the cancer cells.

A study has shown that those provided with black cumin oil as a supplement had a 55 percent increase in T-helper cells function and a 30% boost in natural-killer cell activity.

To conclude, black seed oil showed exceptional promise as a treatment for cancer that doesn't leave a person with the side effects of existing treatments like chemotherapy. The best part is that it is inexpensive and unobtrusive, meaning people who use it as a cancer treatment can go about their routine lives as if nothing has changed.

Chapter # 8: Strengthens the immune system

Immunity in a broader sense includes auto-immune diseases such as cancer, diabetes and migraines. Black cumin has shown the capability to boost the immune system among human beings by 72% in as brief a period of time as a month. Research was performed as early as 1987 by the I.I.M.E.R. to verify the pro-immune system effects of black cumin. These studies showed a marked difference between those administered one gram of black cumin twice daily and the control subjects.

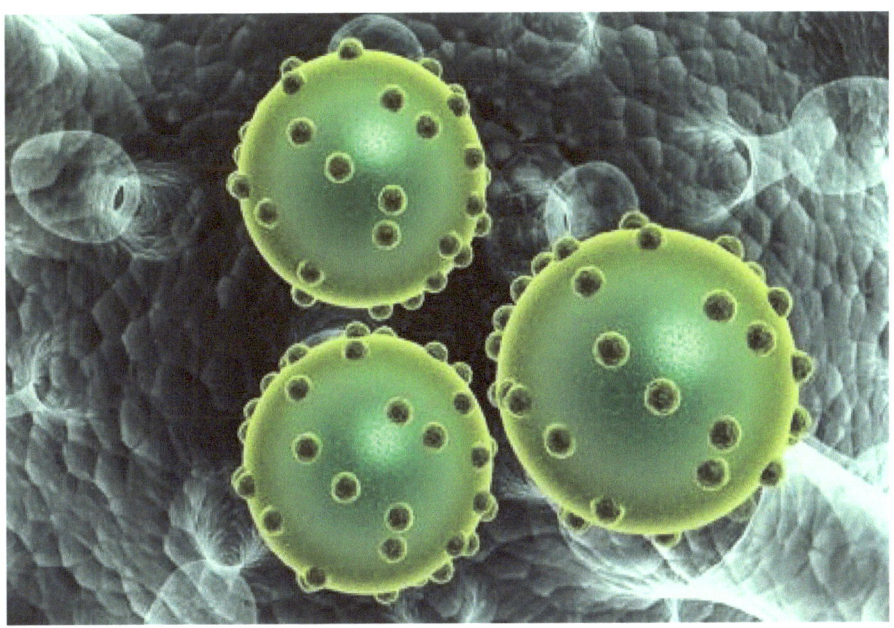

Today, black cumin has become a sustainable treatment for those suffering from auto-immune diseases that are a significant cause of death among the world populace (In 2010, around twenty three and a half million people in America alone were patients coping with auto-immune diseases, eighty of which were deemed as serious health hazards). These auto-immune diseases range from the obscure to those much more prevalent.

Chapter # 9: Alleviates allergic conditions

Allergies are major health problem throughout the world, in particular, the third world countries where adequate medical treatment is unavailable for diseases such as asthma, that cause 200 deaths and over a hundred and fifty thousand hospitalizations among children annually in the U.S. alone. There are many factors which contribute to these allergic conditions including infection, being exposed to allergens, smoke of various types and other environment based pollutants. Additionally, pollen and various foods such as nuts are known to cause allergic reactions in some patients.

Recent studies have pointed to black cumin's allergy alleviating properties – even a small dose of this miraculous seed's oil can be enough to limit the production of allergy inducing chemicals in the body. The active parts of the oil which help fight allergy are thymoquinones and other similar compounds.

Four human studies demonstrated that black cumin oil had the capability to relieve the effects of conditions such as allergic rhinitis, bronchial asthma and atopic eczema. When black seed oil was administered to patients in the four studies, in which the subjects were both adults and children, there was a marked improvement in the way their bodies reacted to the allergies. Allergic rhinitis among children and adults was most notably improved as was the bronchial asthma among children.

A potential explanation for this allergy relieving behavior of black cumin oil can be its effect on the production of leukotrienes and thromboxane. These are compounds that contribute to allergic conditions such bronchial asthma by encouraging inflammatory conditions. The thymoquinone in black cumin oil opposes the reception of leukotriene, as do several other compounds present in it. The exact science behind this opposition lies in the limitation of production of certain compounds, by the black cumin oil, which speed up the synthesis of leukotrienes.

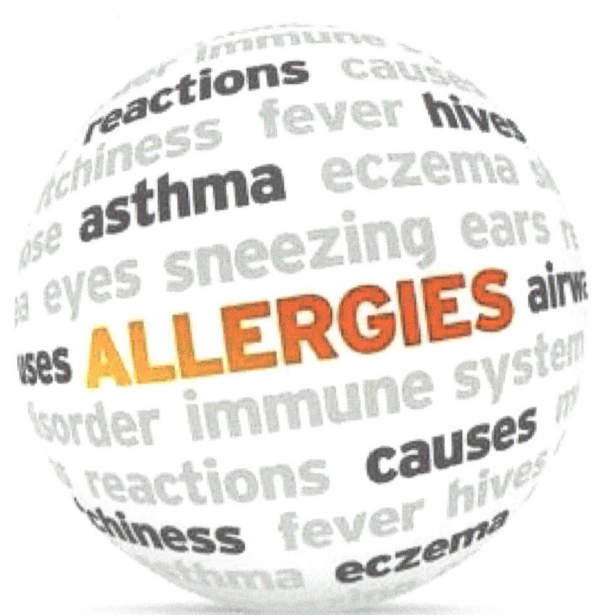

The Arabs were aware of the anti-allergy effects of Black Cumin oil and used it by itself or in a mixture with honey to treat bronchial asthma. A study conducted recently showed that the Arabs were right: Over a three month period, a group of adults was administered black seed, and they should notable improvement in the symptoms of bronchial asthma. Moreover, they became less dependent on their medicines and inhalers.

Chapter # 10: Eases high blood pressure

The humble black cumin seed has also shown the ability to benefit those suffering from high blood pressure.

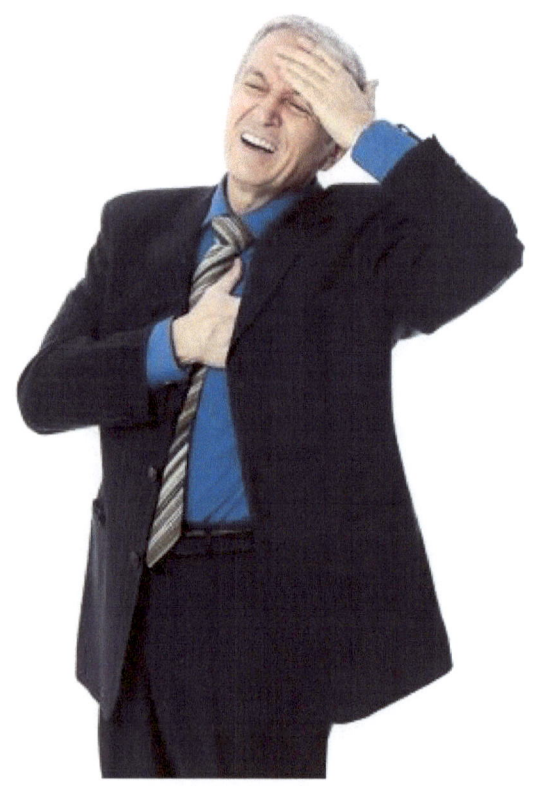

In a research conducted by the Shahrekord University of Medical Sciences in Iran and included in a 2008 edition of the medical journal Fundamental & Clinical Pharmacology, it was seen that those afflicted with mild hypertension i.e. high blood pressure enjoyed improvement in their condition after consuming preset amounts of black cumin extract every day. This improvement was noted two months into the research as the subjects' systolic and diastolic blood pressure was considerably lessened in comparison to those who were the control subjects of the study. There was a correlation between the concentration of the dose and the decrement in blood pressure.

The same study noted a prominent decrease in the subjects' harmful cholesterol levels in contrast with both the levels at the start and with those who were the control. Also, no side effects of the consumption of black cumin extract were observed among the subjects.

Chapter # 11: Counters the effects of radiation

Black seed demonstrated a powerful ability to reduce the effects of exposure to radiation among those being treated by chemotherapy for cancer and those who were exposed to total body irradiation due to some other factors. These effects include neutropenia, reduced neutrophil levels and illness caused due to infections by bacteria and fungi.

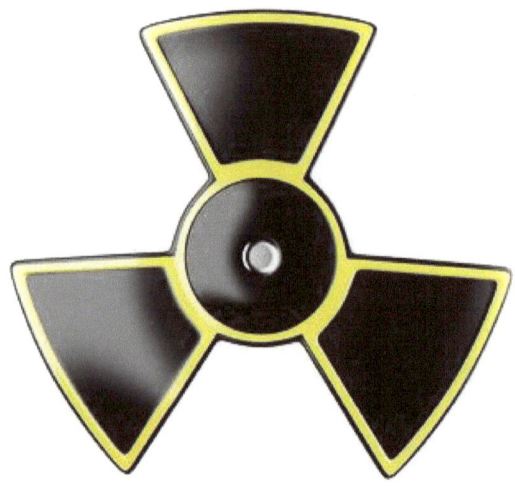

The inflammation caused by exposure to radiation begins to takes it's strain on the individual a few days into radiotherapy, and develops into fibrosis that can take months or even years to expose itself. Research has indicated that the thymoquinone present in black cumin extract possesses anti-inflammatory properties which are why it can be provided to cancer patients being treated with radiotherapy to ease the symptoms of the damage to tissue caused by the radiation.

Several studies have reached the conclusion that black cumin or some form of its extract can be used to allay the effects of radiation including lipid peroxidation, inflammation and toxicity. Because it does not have any side effects of its own, it can safely be administered to those cancer patients who are undergoing severe radiotherapy.

Chapter # 12: Reduces frequency of pediatric seizures

Pediatricians often face the problem of eliminating seizure episodes completely from their patients – a small number of seizures keep occurring in spite of the administration of several drugs to combat the epilepsy.

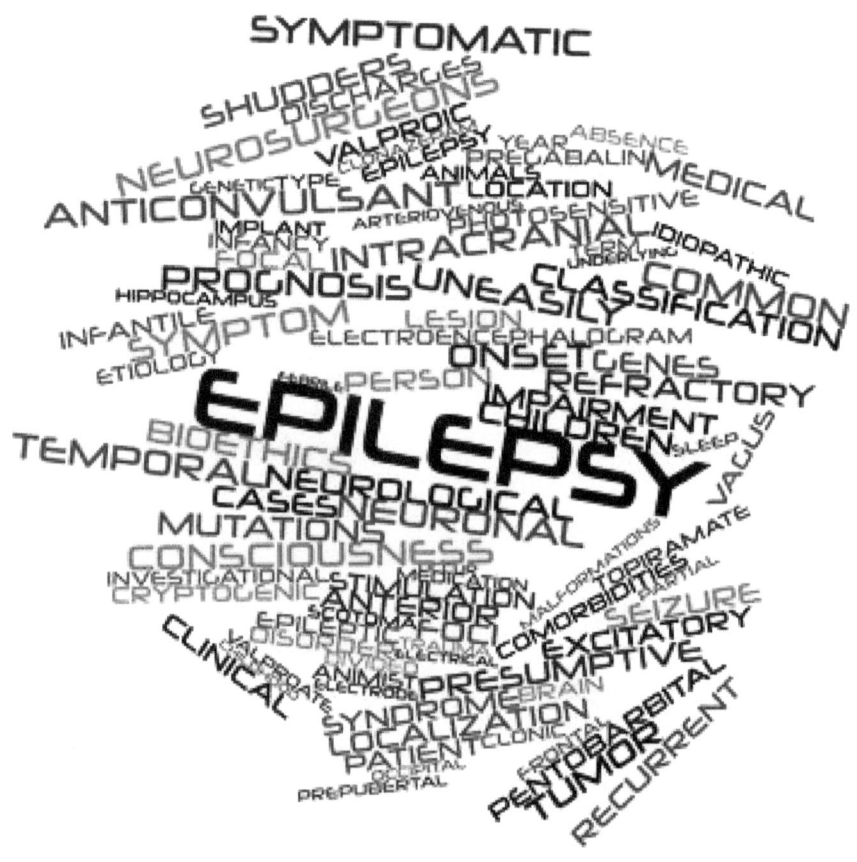

Black cumin has long been known, in folk medicine, as a substance that counters convulsive conditions and this property of black seed has been attributed to the active compound called thymoquinone.

A pilot study was conducted to verify this property of black cumin on a group of children who suffered from refractory epilepsy. After the administration of thymoquinone on some members of the group, the effect on the frequency of their seizures was noted and contrasted with those of the group that formed the control. This was carried out for a month and then a fortnight was provided for the effects of the study to cool down – during the cool down time, they took their usual medicines for the epilepsy and after this time, they were again treated with the thymoquinone for a month. For this period too, the changes in the number of epileptic episodes was noted for each child.

After the conclusion of the pilot study, there was a clear cut reduction in the number of seizures that occurred in the children who were provided with the thymoquinone as compared to those who were given a placebo. Their parents, too, reported more satisfaction with the health of their children.

The study clearly showed that thymoquinone and hence black cumin can be given to children who suffer from intractable epileptic seizures as a way to reduce the frequency of these episodes.

Chapter # 13: Helps in weight loss

Black seed has the property to help you lose weight or keep your weight in check.

An ether extract of black cumin showed the ability to reduce hunger in a study conducted on rats. But this is a promising result which may prove the same effect on humans after further research.

The main mechanism by which black cumin causes you to lose weight is by lowering the level of your blood sugar. Maintenance of blood sugar is essential as not only does it help you lose weight but it also helps in maintaining your overall health.

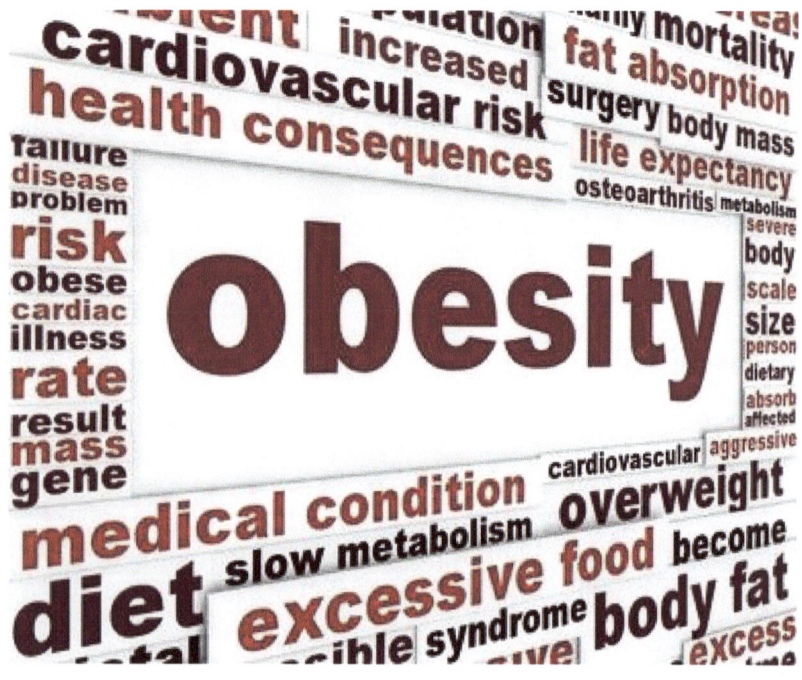

Black cumin contains compounds that help you control your blood sugar by keeping your appetite in check by reducing your desire for excessive carbohydrates. In fact, Shawn Talbot, the writer of 'The Cortisol Connection Diet.', says that by keep your hunger pangs under control, you can lose weight of about two to four lbs. a month without even having to make noticeable changes to your dietary intake.

Proponents of weight loss through black cumin believe that its oil extract is the most efficient form for losing weight. A dose ranging from one to three tablespoons will suffice. Of course, if you find convenient, you may consume it as a seed too.

You should be careful when taking black cumin extract for losing weight, particularly if you're already taking other drugs or herbs to lower your blood glucose levels. If you take it in excess, you may lower your blood sugar levels lower than the recommended threshold which can lead to seizures and unconsciousness among other symptoms e.g. confusion, issues with heartbeat, excessive sweating and problematic vision. This information has been reported by Mayo Clinic.

Chapter # 14: Helps with migraines

Many people try to deal with their migraines by means of over the counter drugs that aren't very light on the wallet and stay at home. They will stay in their room with the shades drawn across the windows and wait for the pain to subside. These drugs may eliminate the temporary causes of the migraine, but be assured – it will return in a week or two, to ruin your day again.

Black cumin, on the other hand, offers a permanent solution to your migraine problem. It's cheap and simple, and does not require any visit to the doctor – you can do it from the comfort of your own home.

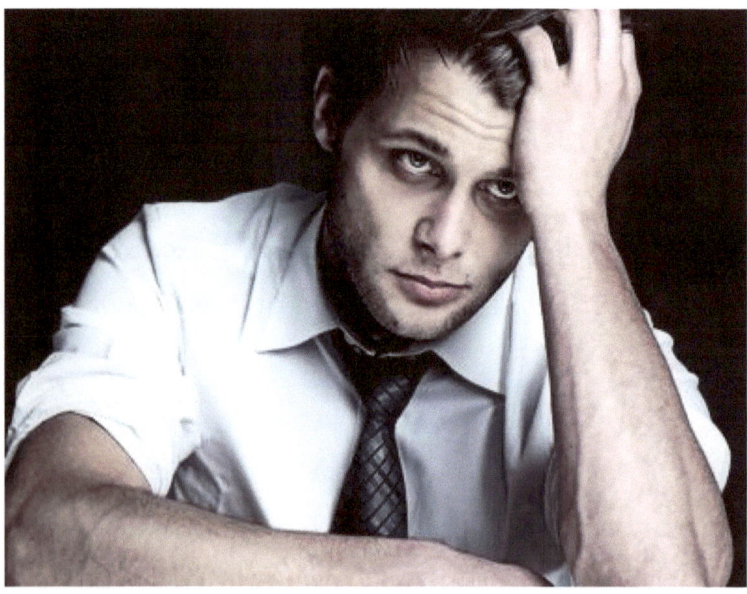

All you have to do is take a dose of nigella sativa as soon as you notice symptoms of a migraine attack. Black cumin comes in two forms – as seeds or as oil – but for migraines, the oil is required by virtue of its concentration. The oil needs to be rubbed behind the head, on the neck; over your eyes and along your hairline. If the top of the head is painful, rub some oil there too. Following this, place a few drops in the nostrils but not too deep. Now inhale the black cumin oil. Do this thrice a day until the headache is cured. After waking up, you should take one tsp. of honey mixed with black cumin, an hour before breakfast. The recipe for a nutritious honey-black cumin mix has been included in the book for your benefit.

Sometimes though, a migraine may not be as harmless as it seems. Should you notice a deviation in the pattern of the headache or any anomalies in its occurrence, it could indicate a serious problem that requires a doctor's consultation. Use black cumin only when your migraine is following a clearly defined pattern.

Conclusion

Now that you've read this book, you'll agree that black cumin is a lot more than that innocent spice it appears to be. Its health benefits had long been recognized in traditional systems of medicine.

It has extremely powerful properties that make it an ideal natural healing agent – it can revitalize the brain, counter cancer, empower the immune system, ease allergic conditions and epilepsy and in a truly astounding feat for such a small plant, it can naturally negate the effects of radiation.

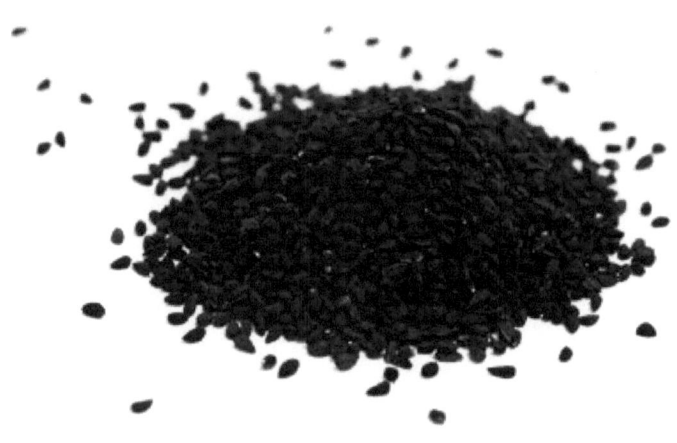

Many people will already be ingesting black cumin in some form routinely – probably in the delicious buns and bread that use it as a topping / garnishing – they will be happy to know that they're not just eating something tasty; they're eating something very healthy. For those who are not, using this spice in their food will definitely be a good idea.

Obviously, there are some precautions to be observed when consuming black cumin, these have been described previously, and the reader will do well to keep them in mind.

Now you should stop reading, and hit the market to buy some of this miraculous, yet extremely inexpensive, seed.

References

1.	http://www.fotolia.com/id/47930241

2.	http://www.fotolia.com/id/50902737

3.	http://www.fotolia.com/id/19784194

4.	http://www.fotolia.com/id/52402197

5.	http://www.fotolia.com/id/51669992

6.	http://www.fotolia.com/id/45156048

7.	http://www.fotolia.com/id/49549245

8.	http://www.fotolia.com/id/59321254

9.	http://www.fotolia.com/id/45257208

10.	http://www.fotolia.com/id/48701190

11.	http://www.fotolia.com/id/45319152

12.	http://www.fotolia.com/id/56739227

13.	http://www.fotolia.com/id/48782829

14.	http://www.fotolia.com/id/50889876

15.	http://www.fotolia.com/id/52425127

Author Bio

Muhammad Usman is a distinguished medical graduate of Allama iqbal medical college (AIMC). He is a professional writer who has been in the field for more than 4 years. During this time he has produced 10,000+ articles, blogs and eBooks on various niches related to diseases, health, fitness, nutrition and well being. He is a regular contributor to several journals related to medicine and surgery. He is the editor of several journals and newspapers.

Download Free Books!

http://MendonCottageBooks.com

Check out some of the other Health Learning Series books

Health Learning Series on Amazon

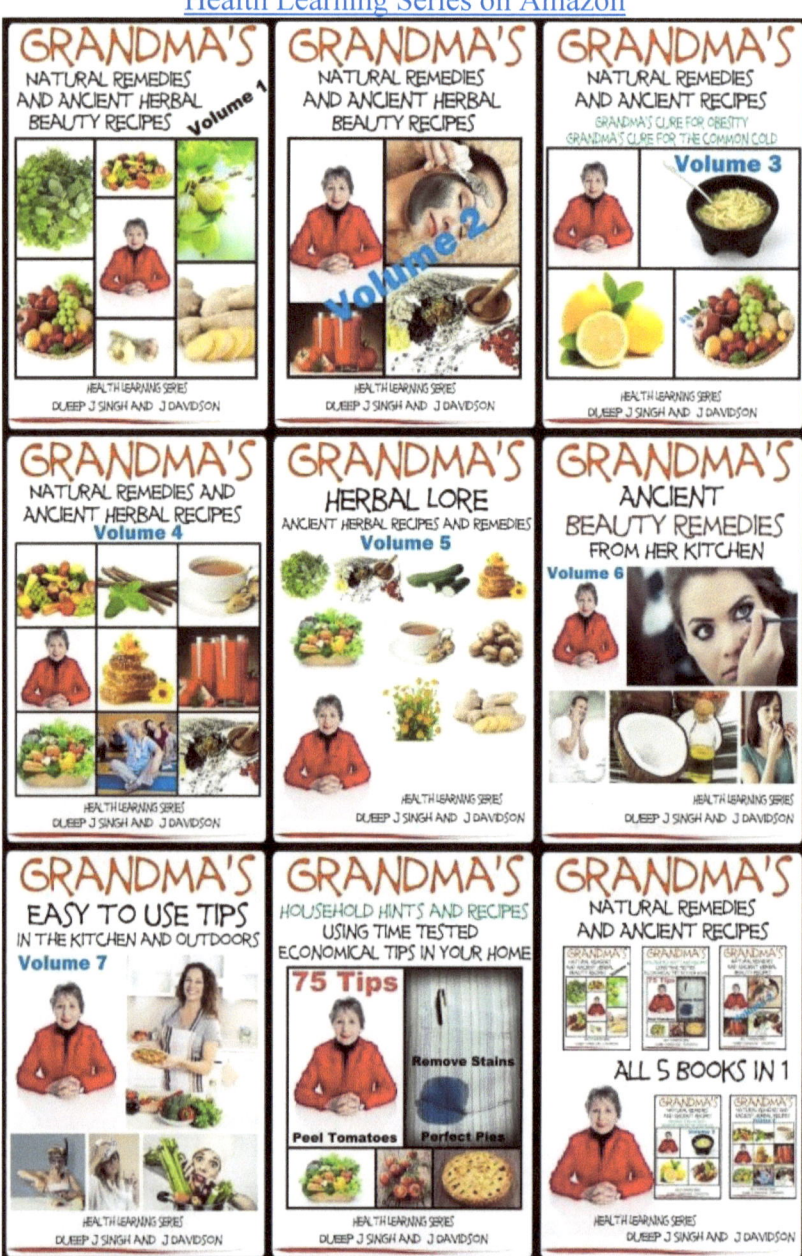

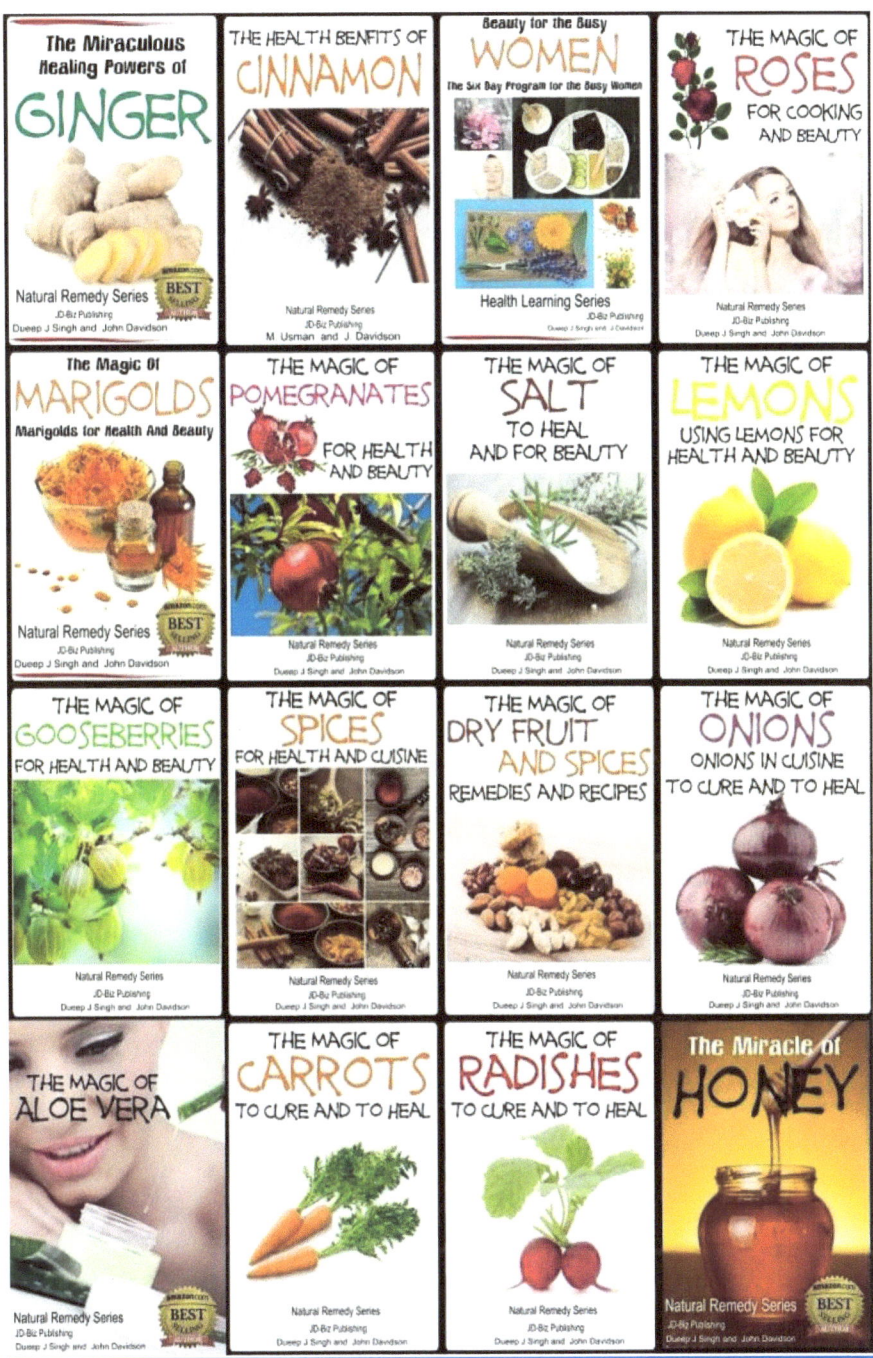

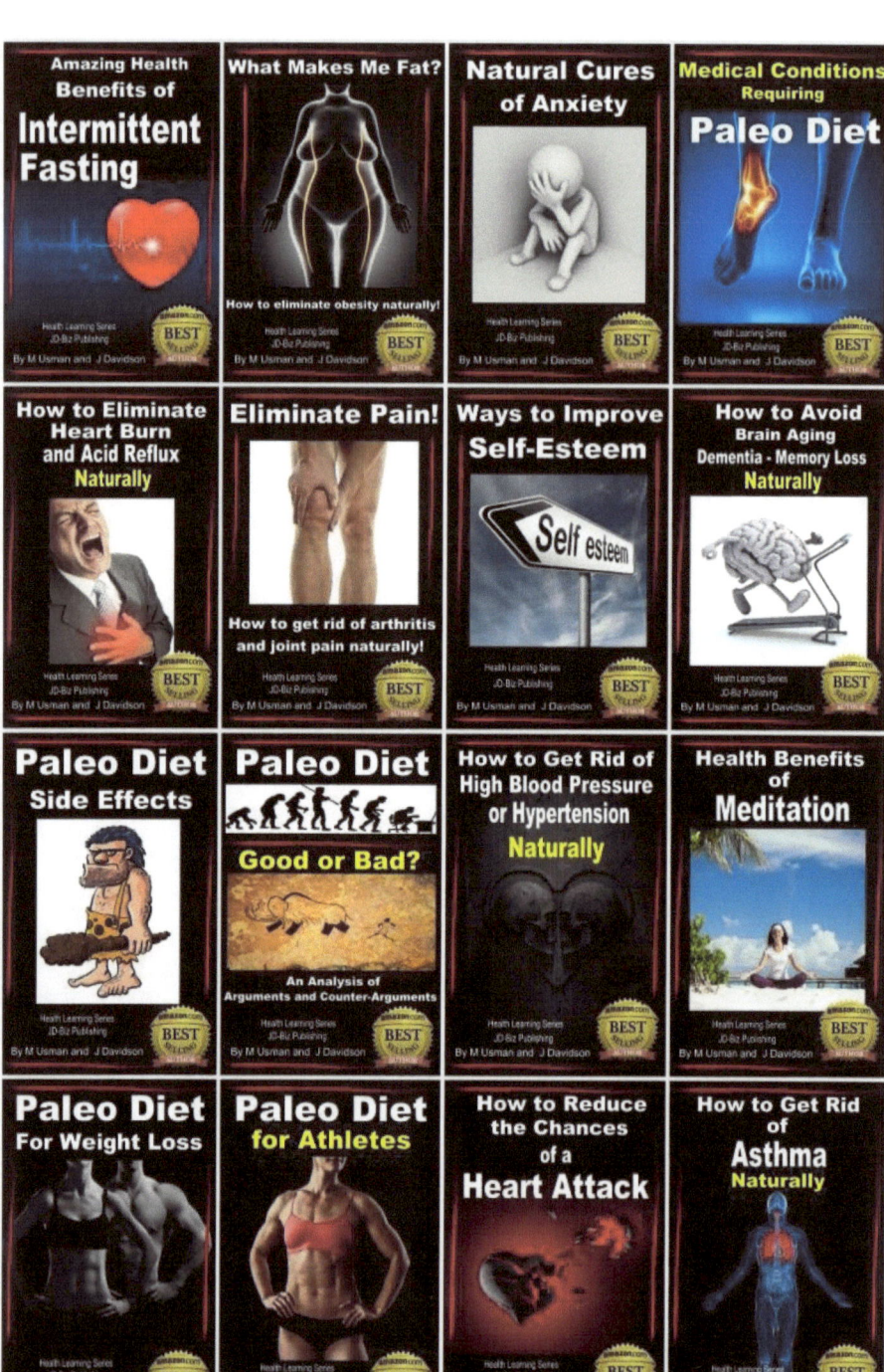

Amazing Animal Books Series

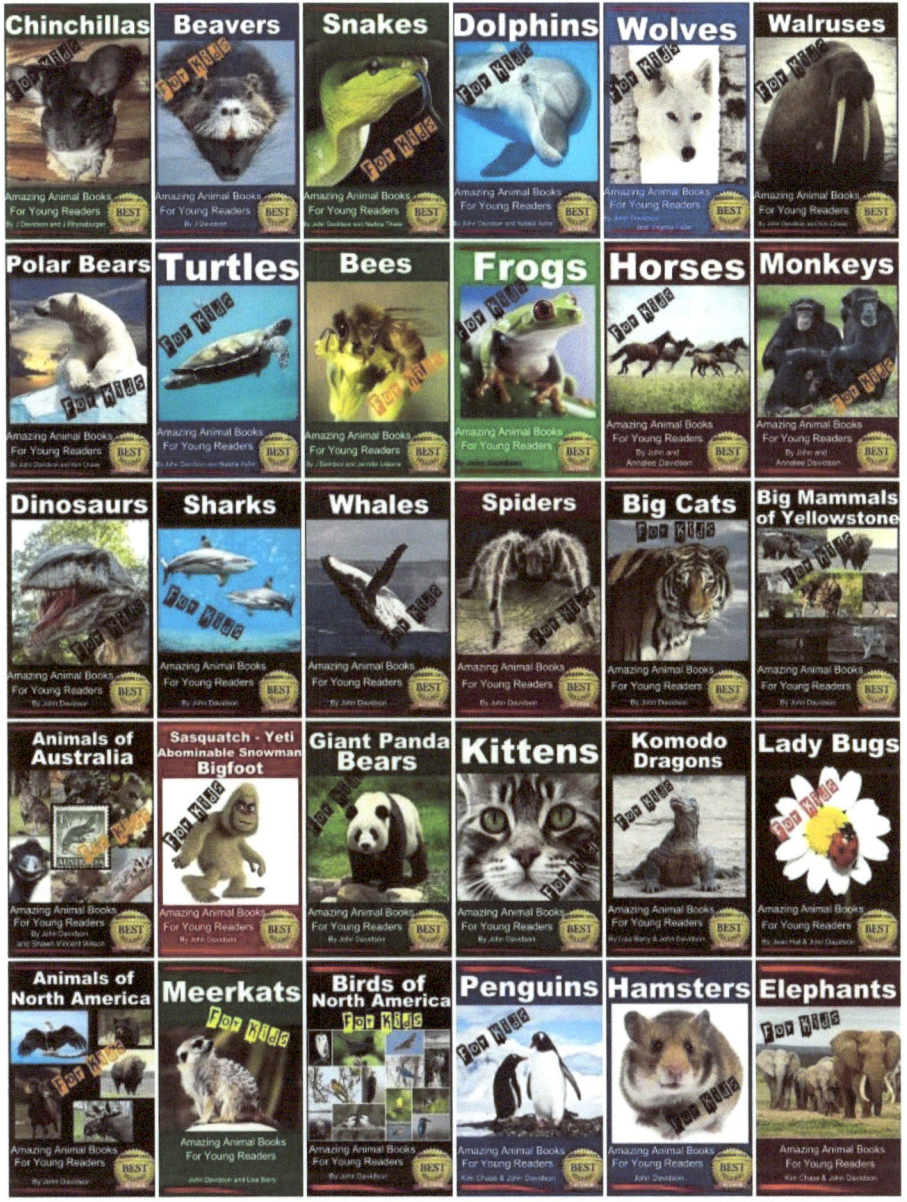

Learn To Draw Series

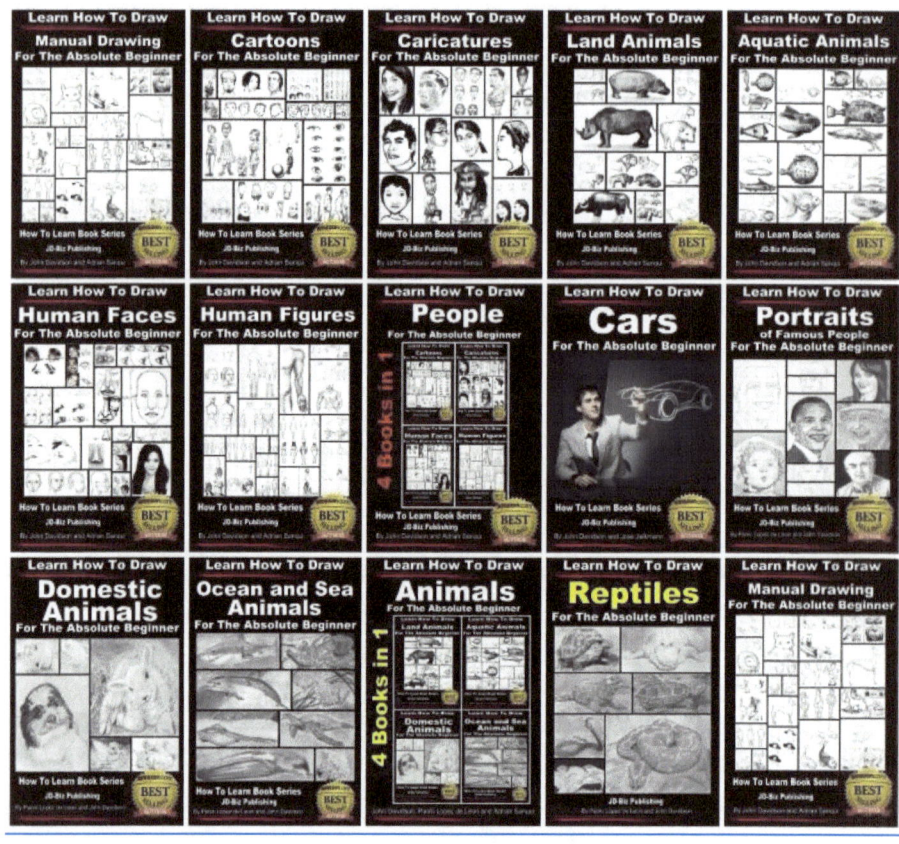

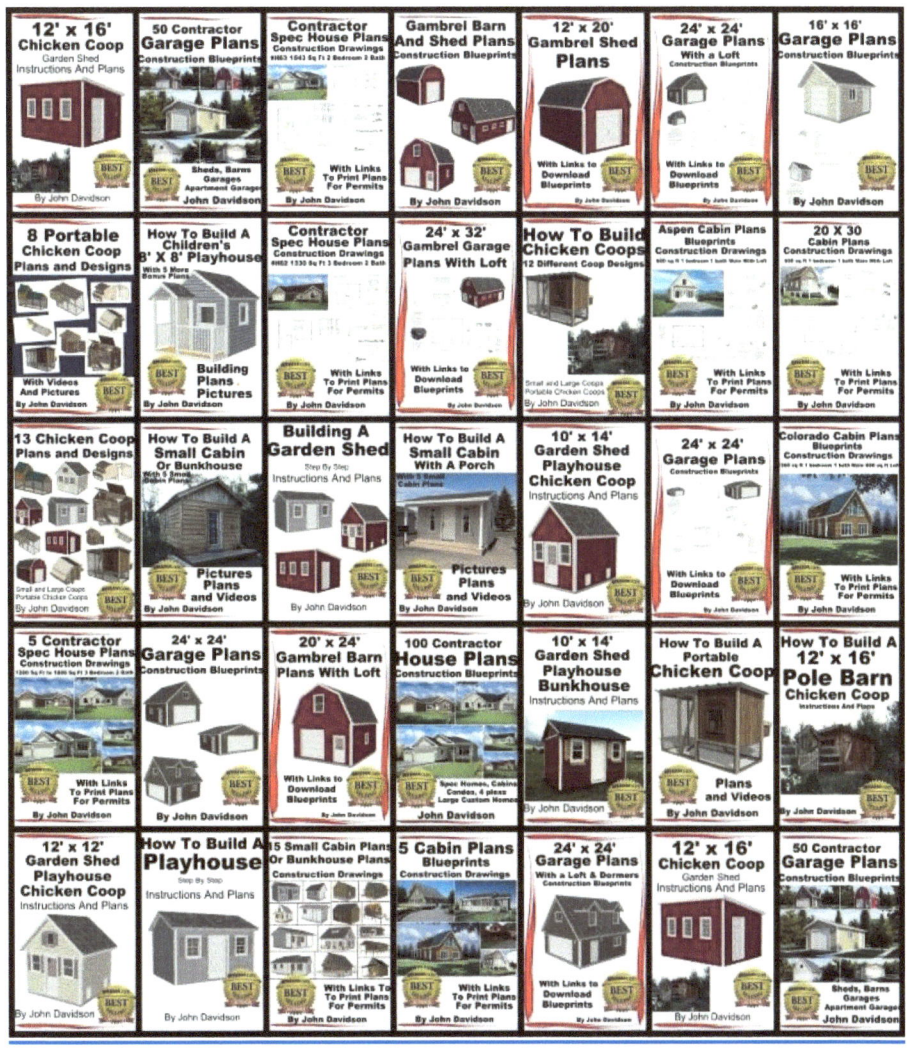

Our books are available at

1. Amazon.com
2. Barnes and Noble
3. Itunes
4. Kobo
5. Smashwords
6. Google Play Books

Download Free Books!

http://MendonCottageBooks.com

Publisher

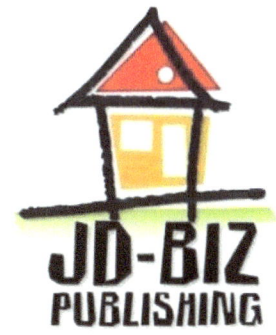

JD-Biz Corp

P O Box 374

Mendon, Utah 84325

http://www.jd-biz.com/

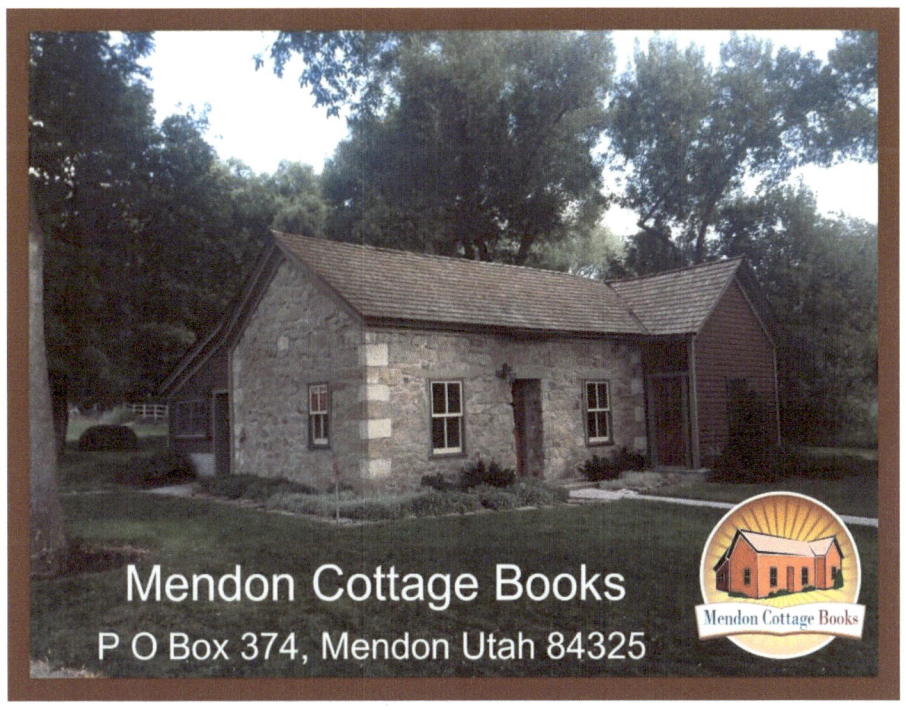

Mendon Cottage Books

P O Box 374, Mendon Utah 84325

www.ingramcontent.com/pod-product-compliance
Lightning Source LLC
Chambersburg PA
CBHW050830290526
45792CB00001B/329